S CHAIR YOGA *for Seniors*

OVER 60

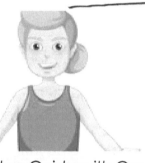
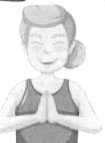

Step by Step Guide with Gentle Exercises to Live Pain-Free & Improve Mobility, Strength, and Flexibility. Maintain Your Independence in Just 10 Minutes Per Day!

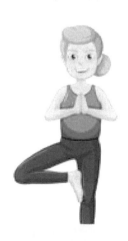
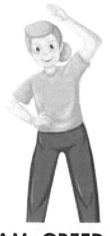
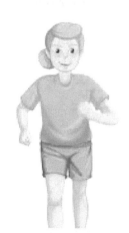

SAM CREED

Table of Contents

INTRODUCTION

Thank you for visiting "Chair Yoga for Seniors: A Comprehensive Guide to Gentle Exercise and Well-Being." This book is intended to introduce seniors over 60 to the great chair yoga practice, offering them a secure and convenient approach to enhancing their physical and mental well-being. This guide will provide step-by-step directions, illustrated postures, and a 10-week training schedule to help you incorporate chair yoga into your daily routine, whether you're new to yoga or have been practicing for years.

In order to promote our general health and vitality as we age, it's crucial to maintain an active lifestyle. However, it could be difficult to engage in typical exercise due to physical restrictions or mobility concerns. In this situation, chair yoga is useful. We may still benefit from yoga without exerting too much stress on our bodies by adjusting poses to be done while seated on a chair. Strength, flexibility, balance, and relaxation can all be improved with the help of the gentle movements, stretches, and breathing exercises found in chair yoga.

There are 15 educational chapters in this book that cover different facets of chair yoga. Each chapter focuses on a distinct subject and offers comprehensive instructions, changes, and advice to guarantee a secure and efficient practice. This guide contains something for everyone, whether you want to increase mindfulness, improve flexibility, relieve stress, or ease joint discomfort.

The book offers a 10-week training schedule that allows you to get started and grow at your own speed by gradually introducing new positions and sequences. You will be guided through each posture with the help of step-by-step instructions and illustrative materials, ensuring perfect alignment and technique. You can also learn how to tailor your chair yoga practice to your particular requirements and tastes.

So sit down, look for a peaceful area, and start on this life-changing journey of self-care and well-being. "Chair Yoga for Seniors" is here to accompany you every step of the journey, whether you're looking for physical health, mental clarity, or just a moment of rest. Let's start investigating chair yoga and learn about all the advantages it has to offer.

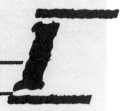

CHAPTER 1

THE ADVANTAGES OF CHAIR YOGA

For seniors over 60, chair yoga is a moderate type of exercise that has several advantages. In this chapter, we shall explore the several benefits of regular chair yoga practice stages. In this chapter, we shall explore the several benefits of regular chair yoga practice. You'll learn all the reasons why chair yoga is such a beneficial exercise, from physical benefits to mental health.

A chair is used to support the body during chair yoga, a modified version of yoga that is performed while sitting on a chair. It is a peaceful, easily accessible activity that has many advantages for people of all ages and skill levels. Chair yoga offers a wonderful opportunity to experience the physical, mental, and emotional advantages of yoga, regardless of whether you have restricted mobility, balance concerns, or simply prefer the comfort of practicing yoga while seated.

Yoga positions, breathing exercises, and meditation practices are all incorporated into chair yoga and modified for seated practice. The emphasis of the exercise is on developing balance, flexibility, strength, and relaxation. It can relax muscle tension, boost circulation, ease joint mobility, lessen stress, and raise general well-being.

Let's thoroughly examine the numerous elements and advantages of chair yoga to offer you a thorough understanding of the technique:

- **Physical Poses:**

Chair yoga poses are made to lengthen and bolster various body areas. The neck, shoulders, arms, back, hips, and legs are all potential targets. Typical chair yoga positions include:

I. Sit tall with your feet flat on the floor in the seated mountain pose. Align your spine and relax your shoulders.

II. Sit tall, hinge forward from your hips, and reach for your feet or shins when performing the seated forward fold.

III. Seated rotation: Holding onto the backrest or armrests for support, sit tall and rotate your upper body to one side.

IV. Seated Warrior II: Create a seated lunge position by sitting tall, extending one leg in front of you, and bending the other knee.

V. Sit tall, placing one foot on the thigh of the person across from you, and bring your hands to your heart. This is the seated tree pose.

- **Exercises for the Breath:**

Chair yoga incorporates conscious breathing as a key component. Exercises that involve deep breathing can soothe anxiety, lower stress levels, and improve the oxygenation of the body. Typical breathing exercises used in chair yoga include:

I. Place your hands on your abdomen, take a deep breath through your nose, and feel your belly rise as you practice abdominal breathing. Feel your tummy lower as you slowly exhale through your nose.

II. Alternate nostril breathing involves sealing off your right nostril with your thumb, taking a breath in through your left nostril, sealing it off with your ring finger, and then exhaling through your right nose. On the opposite side, repeat.

- **Meditation and Relaxation Techniques:**

Meditation and relaxation techniques are included in chair yoga to promote inner tranquility, relaxation, and mental clarity. In chair yoga, some typical methods for concentration and relaxation include:

I. Body Scan Meditation: Focus on various body parts, beginning at your toes and working your way up to your head. Consciously relax any tense or uncomfortable regions that you may have noticed.

II. Close your eyes and picture a tranquil setting, such as a beach or a garden, using guided imagery. Use all of your senses to immerse yourself in the setting.

BENEFITS OF CHAIR YOGA

Seniors and people with restricted mobility can greatly benefit from chair yoga. Some major advantages include:

- Increased Flexibility: Regular chair yoga practice can increase joint flexibility, range of motion, and mobility.
- Strengthening: Chair yoga poses work a variety of muscle groups, enhancing arm, leg, core, and back strength.
- Improved Balance and Stability: Chair yoga postures that involve sitting balance can increase balance and stability and lower the chance of falling.
- Stress Reduction: Breathing exercises and relaxation techniques are incorporated into chair yoga to help people relax and reduce stress.
- Better Posture: By strengthening the core muscles and encouraging perfect alignment, chair yoga helps rectify postural abnormalities.
- Mental Clarity and Focus: Chair yoga's mindfulness and meditation components help enhance one's capacity for concentration, mental clarity, and focus.

- **Improved Circulation:** Chair yoga poses and breathing techniques improve circulation, which is good for the body as a whole.

SAFETY CONSIDERATIONS

Chair yoga is usually considered safe for most people; however, it is still important to practice within your comfort level and get medical advice if you have any particular health conditions or concerns. Adjust positions as necessary, pay attention to your body, and steer clear of any motions that make you hurt or uncomfortable.

The open and adaptable practice of chair yoga may be tailored to suit different needs and skill levels. Homes, elder centers, workplaces, and community centers are just a few venues where it might be used. Regardless of age or physical restrictions, chair yoga offers a gentle and accessible approach to enjoying the benefits of yoga, whether you're a novice or an experienced practitioner.

PHYSICAL ADVANTAGES

Your physical health can improve in a number of ways if you practice chair yoga regularly. You can retain a greater range of motion in your joints as a result of its contribution to flexibility improvement. You'll experience better posture and more flexible muscles by doing mild stretches and motions.

Practicing chair yoga can help you gain muscle. Your core, back, and lower body muscles will get stronger as you practice the seated postures and add weight training. As a result, better stability and balance can lower the risk of falls and injuries.

Chair yoga also enhances joint mobility and wellness. Stretches and moderate motions lubricate the joints, reducing stiffness and soreness. Regular practice can also help manage diseases like osteoporosis and arthritis, bringing about alleviation and enhancing general joint function.

BENEFITS TO THE MIND AND EMOTIONS

The tremendous mental and emotional advantages of chair yoga go beyond its physical advantages. It presents a special chance for stress relief and relaxation. You may relax, clear your thoughts, and find inner peace by using regulated breathing exercises and mindful movements.

Additionally, chair yoga promotes mental clarity and cognitive function. During the practice, you exercise mindfulness, which increases your capacity for concentration and strengthens memory retention. For seniors who want to retain mental acuity and stop cognitive loss, this can be especially helpful.

The emotional state of a person can benefit from chair yoga as well. A sense of self-worth and self-confidence are fostered by the practice, which promotes self-care and self-compassion. It provides a secure environment for emotional exploration and may potentially lessen the effects of despair and anxiety.

Regular chair yoga practice will enable you to enjoy all of these wonderful advantages. In the following chapters, you will be led through a variety of poses and exercises that concentrate on particular areas of development a variety of poses and exercises that concentrate on particular areas of development. When performing chair yoga, keep in mind that consistency is important. Beginning with brief sessions, gradually lengthen and intensify your practice. Chair yoga can enhance your general health and well-being and foster a stronger bond between your body, mind, and spirit if you commit to practicing it regularly.

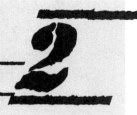

SETTING UP YOUR ENVIRONMENT AND EQUIPMENT

Establishing a welcoming and secure practice area is essential before beginning your chair yoga journey. You will receive instructions on how to set up your practice area and choose the appropriate tools in this chapter. You can improve your chair yoga practice and make sure it goes well by setting up your space and obtaining the necessary equipment.

- **SELECTING THE PROPER SPACE**

Making a welcoming setting for your chair yoga practice depends on choosing the right location. When deciding on your area of practice, keep the following things in mind:

a) Size and Accessibility: Make sure the area is sizable enough to fit your chair and allow for easy movement. It needs to be conveniently reachable and offer enough space for you to freely extend your arms and legs.

b) Lighting: If at all feasible, choose a room with natural light because it can produce a calming atmosphere. Choose a well-lit place or use soft lighting that encourages relaxation and concentration if natural light is scarce.

c) Finding a quiet space where you can practice without interruptions or distractions is important. To reduce disruptions, let family members or roommates know when you practice.

d) Ventilation: When engaging in physical exercise, proper ventilation is crucial. Make sure the area has enough airflow to maintain a comfortable and fresh atmosphere.

- **MAKING SPACE CLEAR AND READY**

It's time to clean up and get ready for the area you've chosen for your chair yoga practice. To create a spotless and welcoming space, take the following actions:

a) Declutter: Clear the area of any extraneous objects, furniture, or obstructions. By clearing the area, you'll have plenty of room to move about and can practice safely.

b) Cleanliness: To create a crisp and inviting atmosphere, dust and clean the area, particularly the floor.

c) A tidy atmosphere helps people focus and fosters a positive attitude.

d) Personal touches: Take into account components that promote calmness and relaxation. This can involve aromatic candles, peaceful art, or plants. Make the area your own to represent your tastes and foster a supportive environment.

- **OBTAINING DEVICES**

Although chair yoga just needs a few pieces of equipment, having the appropriate ones can improve your practice and offer support. Here are some crucial things to think about:

a) A solid chair without arms or with movable armrests is recommended. Make sure the chair is sturdy and able to bear your weight. To prevent slipping, if necessary, put non-slip mats under the chair legs.

b) Cushions and pillows: Depending on your degree of comfort, you might wish to have extra pillows or cushions around to support your knees, hips, or back while performing specific poses. These might add extra comfort and make necessary position modifications.

c) Yoga Mat: While not necessary for chair yoga, a yoga mat can be helpful for sitting activities that require movement or for switching to positions that are performed on the floor. It offers padding and aids in preventing sliding.

d) Blanket: Keep a comfortable blanket close by to serve as a prop for extra support, warmth, or comfort when performing restorative poses or engaging in meditation.

e) Water bottle: During any strenuous exercise, staying hydrated is crucial. Keep a water bottle nearby so you can stay hydrated during practice.

- **CONSIDERATIONS FOR SAFETY**

When doing chair yoga, security should always come first. Observe the following safety measures to create a secure environment:

a) Sturdy Surface: To lessen the chance that your chair will topple over or slip, make sure the floor beneath it is level and sturdy. Practice areas that are slick or uneven should be avoided.

b) Correct Alignment: When performing postures, pay attention to how your body is positioned. With your shoulders relaxed and your spine stretched, sit tall. Avoid any uncomfortable movements that require effort or force.

c) Modifications and Props: Adjust poses to your body's capabilities and limitations as necessary. Use props to support your body and preserve good posture, such as cushions or pillows.

d) Pay Attention to Your Body: Respect the requirements and limitations of your body. A stance or movement should be modified or avoided if it causes pain or discomfort. Work within your comfort zone and respect your body's boundaries.

Setting up a comfortable setting for your chair yoga practice requires taking important measures like organizing your area and obtaining the required supplies. You can create a tranquil environment that encourages focus and relaxation by choosing a suitable location, tidying the room, and adding your own touches. Having the appropriate tools, such as a comfortable chair, cushions, and props, ensures your practice is both safe and comfortable. Always put safety first, pay attention to your body, and adjust as necessary. You are prepared to start your chair yoga adventure with confidence and enjoyment if you have a suitable place and the necessary equipment.

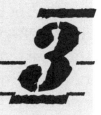

EXERCISES TO WARM UP FOR CHAIR YOGA

Exercises that warm up your body are crucial before doing chair yoga. They ensure a safe and successful session by promoting blood circulation, warming up your muscles, and loosening your joints. We'll walk you through a number of easy warm-up exercises in this chapter that you may work into your chair yoga regimen.

- **Neck Rolls:**

Neck rolls are performed while sitting tall in a chair with the feet flat on the floor. Roll your head in a clockwise circle and gently tuck your chin toward your chest. Take your time and move in a smooth, fluid motion. Roll your head clockwise for a few rotations, then counterclockwise. This exercise increases mobility and relieves neck stress.

- **Shoulder Rolls:**

Rolling your shoulders back will help them become more relaxed and move away from your ears. Exhale as you move your shoulders back and down after inhaling while raising them up toward your ears. To perform many shoulder rolls, alternating between forward and backward rotations. Shoulder rolls aid in easing stress and enhancing shoulder joint flexibility.

- **Arm Circles:**

With your palms facing down, extend your arms out to the sides at shoulder height. Start gently circling your arms, progressively enlarging the size of the circles. Change the circles' directions after a few revolutions. The shoulder joints are warmed up during this workout, and the arms' muscles are also activated.

- **Spinal Twist:**

Place your feet firmly on the ground while sitting upright in your chair. Put your left hand on the back of the armrest and your right hand on the outside of your left leg. Take a deep breath in and, as you let it out, gently twist your torso to the left with the help of your hands. For a few breaths, hold the twist while sensing the little stretch in your spine. On the other side, repeat. The spinal twist relieves back strain while also enhancing spinal mobility.

- **Rotations of the wrist and ankle:**

Extend your right leg in front of you, heel firmly planted. Rotate your ankle slowly and steadily in both clockwise and counterclockwise directions. The same rotations should be done with your left ankle. Next, extend your arms out in front of you while rotating your wrists in a clockwise and counterclockwise motion. The often-overlooked ankles and wrists are made more mobile and flexible by these exercises.

Your body will be better prepared for chair yoga practice thanks to these warm-up movements, which will also improve your flexibility and lower your chance of injury. Keep in mind to move slowly and deliberately, being aware of your body's sensations. After warming up, let's continue on to Chapter 4, where we'll examine seated positions for flexibility and strength.

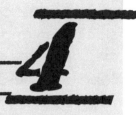

CHAPTER 4

SEATED POSES FOR STRENGTH AND FLEXIBILITY

In this chapter, we'll look at several seated positions with the goal of increasing flexibility and strength. These poses are suitable for seniors over 60 because they may be completed completely from the comfort of your chair. Always pay attention to your body and adjust the poses as necessary to meet your unique requirements and capabilities.

- **Seated Mountain Pose (Tadasana):**

Sit tall in Tadasana (seated mountain pose), placing your hands on your thighs and your feet flat on the floor. As you ground yourself in the here and now, close your eyes and take a few deep breaths. Think of a cord stretching your spine by tugging your head's crown upward. This position enhances alignment throughout the body and posture.

- **Seated Forward Fold (Paschimottanasana):**

Sit at the edge of your chair with your feet hip-width apart in the seated forward fold position

(Paschimottanasana). Exhale as you bend forward from your hips and extend your hands toward the floor or your feet after inhaling to lengthen your spine. You can wrap a strap over your feet and grip onto it for support if you have restricted flexibility. The lower back, shoulders, and hamstrings are all stretched in this position.

- **Seated Spinal Twist (Ardha Matsyendrasana):**

Place your feet firmly on the ground while seated sideways on your chair. Take a deep breath in to stretch your spine, then let it out as you twist toward the back of the chair with one hand on the back of the seat and the other on your outer thigh. Hold the twist for a few breaths while feeling your spine gently rotate. On the opposite side, repeat. This position enhances digestion and spinal flexibility.

- **Seated Warrior Pose (Virabhadrasana):**

Sit tall with your feet spread apart in the seated warrior pose (Virabhadrasana). Keep your left foot pointed ahead while turning your right foot out. Take a deep breath and lift your arms aloft while keeping them parallel to the floor. Breathe out as you flex your right knee, making sure it stays in line with your ankle. Repeat on the opposite side after holding the position for a few breaths. The seated warrior pose enhances balance while strengthening the legs and stretching the inner thighs.

- **Seated Cat-Cow Pose:**

Sit in the cat-cow position with your hands on your thighs and your feet flat on the floor. Take a deep breath in and arch your spine into the cow pose by pulling your shoulder blades together and elevating your chest. In the "Cat Pose," you circle your spine as you exhale, tucking your chin into your chest and pulling your belly button up toward your spine. Continue to alternate between these two poses while controlling your breathing to produce a soft movement that relaxes the spine.

- **Seated Pigeon Pose:**

Sit upright with your feet flat on the floor in the seated pigeon pose. Forming a figure-four, place your right ankle on top of your left leg. In order to protect your knee, flex your right foot. To intensify the stretch, if it feels comfortable, you might lightly press down on your right knee. Repeat on the opposite side after holding the position for a few breaths. Stretching the hips and glutes while seated in a pigeon pose helps increase flexibility in these areas.

- **Seated Eagle Arms (Garudasana):**

Sit tall with your feet level on the floor. Raise your arms to shoulder height in front of you. Bring your hands together as you cross your right arm across your left arm. Put your forearms together if you can, then point your fingertips upward. If this is difficult, just give your shoulders a simple arm embrace. After a few breaths, hold the position and then alternate crossing your arms. The shoulders and upper back are stretched while seated, improving flexibility and relieving stress.

These seated poses have the potential to increase both flexibility and strength. Include them in your chair yoga regimen by starting with a short period of time in each pose and extending it as you get more comfortable. Keep in mind to breathe slowly and steadily throughout the practice. We'll discuss gentle stretches to reduce muscle tension in the following chapter.

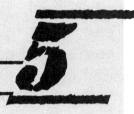

CHAPTER 5

GENTLE STRETCHES TO EASE MUSCLE TENSION ARE COVERED

We will explore a number of easy stretches in this chapter that are intended to ease stress and promote relaxation. These stretches are doable and advantageous for seniors over 60 because they can be done while seated in a chair. Always pay attention to your body, be aware of your limitations, and adjust the positions as necessary.

- **Neck Stretch**

Stretch your neck by sitting tall and slowly pushing your right ear toward your right shoulder. Your neck's left side ought to feel somewhat stretched. Repeat the stretch on the other side after holding it for a few breaths. Observe any discomfort and modify the range of motion as necessary. This stretching exercise focuses on the neck muscles, relieving stress and enhancing flexibility.

- **Shoulder and Upper Back Stretch**

Straighten your right arm in front of you so that it is parallel to the ground to stretch your shoulders and upper back. Feeling a stretch in the back of your shoulder, place your left hand behind your right elbow and slowly bring the right arm towards your chest. After holding for a few breaths, switch to the opposite side. The tension in the shoulders and upper back is relieved by this stretch.

- **Chest Opener**

Interlace your fingers behind your back with your palms facing inward as a chest opener. Allowing your chest to expand, straighten your arms, and slowly elevate them away from your body. As your shoulders and chest extend, take a few deep breaths. If you find it difficult to maintain this grasp, you can hold onto a strap, a towel, or the chair's sides. This stretch helps with posture and eases chest strain to offset the consequences of prolonged sitting and hunching.

- **Sitting Side Bend**

Maintain a straight posture while reaching to the left side with your right arm raised overhead. Feel the stretch down the right side of your body as you gently tilt your torso to the left. Avoid putting any tension on your neck by keeping both hips firmly planted on the chair. After a few breaths of holding, switch sides. By lengthening the muscles on either side of your body, you can increase flexibility and reduce stiffness.

- **Sitting Forward Fold Variation**

Place your feet hip-width apart and sit at the edge of your chair. Your arms should be out in front of you, palms outward. Interlace your fingers. Exhale as you fold forward from your hips, allowing your arms to come overhead and your head to relax. Inhale to lengthen your spine. As your shoulders, hamstrings, and lower back stretch, take a few slow, deep breaths. The entire rear body can be gently released with this version.

- **Seated Calf Stretch**

Stretch your calves while seated by extending your right leg in front of you while keeping your heel on the floor. You should feel a stretch in your calf muscle as you flex your right foot and softly bring the sole of your foot close to your torso. After holding for a few breaths, switch to the opposite side. The calf muscles, which might tighten from prolonged sitting or inactivity, are the focus of this stretch.

- **Sitting Figure-Four Stretch**

Keep your feet flat on the floor while sitting tall. Make a figure-four by crossing your right ankle over your left thigh. Feel a stretch in your right hip as you softly press down on your right knee. After holding for a few breaths, switch to the opposite side. This stretch focuses on the hip muscles, releasing tension and enhancing hip mobility.

These simple stretches provide a calming and therapeutic method for reducing tension in the muscles and encouraging relaxation. Utilize them as part of your chair yoga routine, taking your time to discover a relaxing stretch that works for your body. In each stretch, keep your focus on your breathing and deepen it. We'll look at chair yoga positions for better balance and posture in the following chapter.

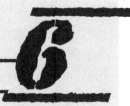

CHAPTER

CHAIR YOGA POSES TO IMPROVE POSTURE AND BALANCE

It's essential to keep your posture and balance in check to be healthy overall and avoid falling. We'll look at some chair yoga postures in this chapter that are intended to strengthen the core, improve posture, and improve balance. These positions can be done with the assistance of a chair and are appropriate for seniors over 60.

- **Seated Mountain Pose (Tadasana):**

Start in the seated mountain pose, or tadasana, by sitting tall, placing your feet firmly on the floor, and placing your hands on your thighs. In order to stretch your spine, ground through your sit bones and picture a cord dragging your head's crown up towards the ceiling. Keep your breath calm and your core muscles contracted. This position encourages optimal alignment and lays the groundwork for improved posture and balance.

- **Seated High Mountain Pose:**

Inhale as you raise your arms aloft with your palms facing each other in the seated mountain pose. Then, visualize raising your fingertips while lengthening your spine. Keep your posture strong and upright by engaging your core. As you reach upward, notice how your sides are being stretched. Release your arms after holding the position for a few breaths. The High Mountain Pose, when seated, strengthens the core and enhances posture.

- **Sitting Spinal Extension:**

Sit tall, with your feet level on the floor, and place your hands on your thighs. Draw a deep breath in, stretch your spine, softly arch your back, and lift your chest upward. Open your heart and tuck your shoulder blades together. After exhaling for a few breaths, release the pose and return to a neutral position. This position encourages a more upright posture and works to prevent the effects of slouching.

- **Twist while seated:**

Place your feet firmly on the floor and lean back in your chair. Take a deep breath in to stretch your spine, then let it out as you twist toward the back of the chair with one hand on the back of the seat and the other on your outer thigh. As you intensify the twist, keep your core engaged and your spine straight. Repeat on the opposite side after holding the position for a few breaths.

The seated twist increases spinal mobility and fortifies the balance-maintaining core muscles.

- **Seated Tree Pose (Vrksasana):**

Sit tall in the tree pose (Vrksasana), your feet flat on the floor. Lift your right foot off the ground and shift your weight to your left foot. Find a position that feels secure and comfortable for you, and place the sole of your right foot on your left inner thigh or calf. Alternatively, raise your arms above your head or bring your hands to your heart. Maintain your equilibrium and a steady gaze. After a few breaths, hold the position and then exchange sides. Balance is improved, leg muscles are strengthened, and attention is enhanced in the seated tree pose.

- **Sitting Leg Extension:**

Keep your feet flat on the floor while sitting tall. Engage your thigh muscles as you extend your right leg forward, parallel to the ground. Hold the position with your right foot extended for a few breaths. Repeat with the left leg after lowering your right leg. Leg muscles are strengthened and stability is increased with seated leg extensions.

Sitting Cat-Camel Pose: Sit with your hands on your thighs and your feet flat on the floor. In the "Cow Pose," inhale as you elevate your chest and let your belly drop while arching your back. When you exhale, assume the cat pose by arching your back, tucking your chin into your chest, and pulling your belly button in against your spine. With your breath, alternate between these two positions as you keep your body firm and in balance. The seated cat-camel pose develops the core muscles necessary for healthy posture while improving spinal flexibility.

These chair yoga positions concentrate on improving posture and balance. Practice them thoughtfully, focusing on good posture and using the required muscles. Adding these postures to your practice on a regular basis can boost stability, enhance posture, and improve your general sense of well-being. We shall concentrate on chair yoga for relaxation and stress reduction in the following chapter.

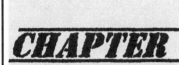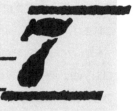

CHAPTER 7

CHAIR YOGA FOR STRESS REDUCTION

Finding time to unwind and reduce stress in today's hectic environment is crucial for our health. In this chapter, we'll look at some breathing exercises and chair yoga positions that can help you unwind and reduce tension. These easy exercises may be done anywhere, at any time, and they offer a tranquil haven in the middle of daily stress.

- **Seated Forward Fold (Paschimottanasana):**

Sit at the edge of your chair with your feet hip-width apart in the seated forward fold position (Paschimottanasana). When you exhale, tilt forward from your hips and extend your hands toward the floor or your feet. Take a deep breath and stretch your spine. Relax your neck and head by doing so. In this forward fold, take calm, deep breaths and feel the tension in your shoulders and back melt away. After holding the position for a few breaths, slowly stand back up.

- **Seated Heart Opener:**

Sit tall, feet flat on the floor, and place your hands on your thighs for the seated heart opener. Take a deep breath in and gradually arch your upper back as you exhale. This will bring your shoulder blades together and widen your chest. Allow your breath to be unrestricted as you raise your heart to the sky. Hold this heart-opening stance for a few moments while taking deep breaths to feel open and relaxed.

- **Seated Neck and Shoulder Release:**

Sit tall and let your shoulders fall while performing a seated neck and shoulder release. Deeply inhale, then, as you exhale, tuck your right ear up against your right shoulder so that your left side of the neck is stretched. As you stretch deeper, place your right hand on the left side of your head and softly press down. After a few breaths spent stretching thoroughly, switch sides. This pose encourages relaxation by easing tension in the shoulders and neck.

- **Seated Belly Breathing:**

Sit comfortably with your feet flat on the floor and your hands on your tummy while belly breathing. Take a few long, deep breaths while focusing on your belly. Then close your eyes. Allowing your belly to rise and expand as you inhale and feeling it gently contract as you exhale. Spend many minutes doing this deep belly breathing, concentrating just on the breath. The relaxation response is triggered, and the nervous system is calmed by this technique.

- **Seated Half-Spinal Twist:**

Place your feet firmly on the floor and lean sideways in your chair. Take a deep breath in to stretch your spine, then let it out as you twist toward the back of the chair with one hand on the back of the seat and the other on your outer thigh. As you gently twist, close your eyes, and inhale deeply. With each breath, sense the removal of stress and tension. After a few breaths, hold the twist and then switch sides.

- **Seated Meditation:**

Sit comfortably in your chair for seated meditation, keeping your spine straight and your body at ease. Your hands should be in your lap or on your thighs. Close your eyes gently and focus on your breathing. Allow your breath's natural rhythm to lead you into a profound level of relaxation as you pay attention to it. Simply acknowledge your ideas as they come and go, bringing your attention back to the breath. Spend as much time as you like in this seated meditation, allowing yourself to feel a sense of peace and tranquility inside.

These breathing exercises and chair yoga poses offer a haven of tranquility and aid in stress reduction. Include them in your routine every day, especially when you need to relax and achieve inner calm. A better sense of relaxation, mental clarity, and general wellbeing will develop with regular practice. We shall examine chair yoga poses for joint flexibility and mobility in the following chapter.

CHAPTER 8

CHAIR YOGA POSE FOR JOINT FLEXIBILITY AND MOBILITY

Seniors must maintain joint flexibility and mobility to increase their overall range of motion and avoid stiffness. This chapter will go through some chair yoga poses that are designed to increase flexibility and joint mobility. Your joints will stay flexible thanks to these mild activities, which also encourage healthy aging.

- **Seated Ankle Rolls:**

Sit upright with your feet flat on the floor and perform seated ankle rolls. Gently spin your ankle in a circle, first in one direction and then the other, while lifting your right foot. Ankle rolls should be done a few times before switching to the left foot. This exercise increases ankle mobility and lessens ankle stiffness.

- **Seated Knee Lifts:**

Sit tall with your feet flat on the floor and perform seated knee lifts. While keeping your right knee bent, lift your right foot a few inches off the floor. After maintaining the posture for a few breaths, bring your foot back down. On the left, repeat. This exercise improves flexibility in the knee joints and strengthens the muscles surrounding the knees.

- **Hip circles while seated:**

Place your feet firmly on the floor and lean back in your chair. Put your hands on your hips and start moving your hips in a circular motion. Increase the size of the circles gradually after beginning with smaller ones. Change to the opposite direction after a few rotations in one direction. This motion encourages hip joint mobility and reduces hip stiffness.

- **Sitting Spinal Twist:**

Ensure that your feet are planted firmly on the ground. Take a deep breath in and, as you let it out, twist your torso to the right, putting your right hand on the chair's backrest and your left hand on the outside of your right leg. With each exhalation, progressively deepen the twist while maintaining spinal length. After a few breaths of holding the twist, come back to the middle and repeat on the left side. This position increases flexibility in the spine and improves spinal motion.

- **Seated Shoulder Rolls:**

Sit tall with your feet flat on the floor and your hands resting on your thighs for seated shoulder rolls. Exhale while rolling your shoulders back and down after inhaling while raising them up toward your ears. Perform a few rounds of shoulder rolls while being conscious of your movements and allowing them to be easy and natural. This exercise encourages shoulder joint mobility and relieves shoulder stress.

- **Seated Wrist Stretches:**

Stretch your wrists while seated by extending your arms in front of you, palms down. Rotate your wrists slowly in a circle, first in one direction and then the other. Feel your wrists and forearms gently stretch. Stretch your wrists several times, then let your arms rest. This exercise increases the flexibility and mobility of the wrist.

- **Seated Neck and Head Tilts:**

Sit tall with your feet flat on the floor to avoid neck and head tilts while seated. Take a deep breath in, and then, as you exhale, lower your chin so that it stretches the back of your neck. After a few breaths in this position, carefully raise your head back to the middle. Repetition of the motion with a head tilt to the right will cause a stretch along the left side of your neck. Hold for a few breaths before transferring to the other side. These slight head and neck tilts increase neck mobility and reduce neck muscular stress.

You can move more easily and maintain a greater degree of comfort in your everyday activities by practicing these chair yoga postures on a regular basis, which will assist in enhancing joint mobility and flexibility. Always practice the poses attentively, paying attention to your body's limitations and changing as necessary.

We will concentrate on chair yoga for strength and stability in the following chapter.

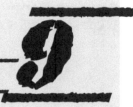

CHAPTER

CHAIR YOGA FOR STRENGTH AND STABILITY

Seniors must maintain their strength and stability to support their everyday activities and lower their risk of falling. We will look at several chair yoga postures in this chapter that work on different muscle groups and improve overall strength and stability. These postures can be performed safely and successfully, giving a strong foundation for practical movement and increased self-assurance.

- **Leg press while seated:**

Stand tall with your feet flat on the floor. For support, put your hands on the chair's sides. Take a deep breath in and, as you exhale, plant your right foot firmly to work your right leg muscles. After a few breaths of holding, release. On the left, repeat. This exercise enhances lower body strength and stability by strengthening the quadriceps, hamstrings, and calf muscles.

- **Seated Row:**

Hold on to the chair's sides while sitting up straight, your feet flat on the floor, and your arms out in front of you. Squeeze your upper back muscles by taking a deep breath in and then, as you exhale, draw your shoulder blades together and pull your elbows back. Hold for a short while, then let go. This exercise strengthens the upper back muscles while enhancing stability and posture.

- **Seated Bicep Curl:**

With your feet level on the floor and your arms extended side by side with your palms facing forward, perform a seated bicep curl. As you exhale, bend your elbows and bring your hands up to your shoulders. Take a big breath vol on the floor and your arms extended side by side with your palms facing forward, perform a seated bicep curl. As you exhale, bend your elbows and bring your hands up to your shoulders. Take a big breath. Use your bicep muscles and keep your elbows close to your torso. Hold for a little while before gradually bringing your hands back down. This exercise increases arm strength and stability while strengthening the biceps.

- **Seated Chest Press:**

With your feet flat on the floor and your hands resting on your thighs, perform a seated chest press. As you exhale, thrust your hands forward and raise your arms in front of you. Take a deep breath. Imagine pressing against resistance while contracting your chest muscles. Hold for a short while, then let go. This exercise strengthens the chest muscles and improves the stability and strength of the upper body.

- **Sitting Core Twist:**

Ensure that your feet are firmly planted on the ground. Hold onto the chair's sides or place your hands on your hips for support. Deeply inhale, then, while exhaling, turn your torso to the right while contracting your abdominal muscles. Hold for a short while before going back to the middle. On the left, repeat. This exercise enhances core stability while strengthening the oblique muscles.

- **Seated Glute Squeeze:**

Squeeze your glutes while seated and keep your feet flat on the floor. Squeeze your glute muscles as you exhale, elevating your hips a little bit off the chair. Hold for a short while, then let go. This exercise strengthens and stabilizes the hips by focusing on the gluteal muscles.

- **Seated Shoulder Press:**

Press your shoulders while seated by sitting tall, placing your feet flat on the floor, and extending your arms in front of you with your palms facing forward. Take a deep breath in and, as you exhale, raise your hands and arms high. Consider pressing against resistance while tensing your shoulder muscles. Hold for a little while before gradually bringing your hands back down. This exercise increases upper-body strength and stability while strengthening the shoulder muscles.

By including these chair yoga postures in your practice, you may improve your strength and stability, which will help you move more confidently and maintain your independence during daily activities. Always pay attention to your body and adjust the poses as necessary. We shall discuss chair yoga for energy and vigor in the following chapter.

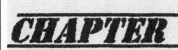 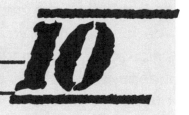

CHAIR YOGA FOR ENERGY AND VITALITY

In order to completely enjoy their daily lives, seniors must feel invigorated and bright. In this chapter, we'll look at a number of chair yoga positions and breathing exercises that work to increase energy and vitality. You can add these energizing rituals to your daily routine to feel more awake, aware, and refreshed.

- **Seated Mountain Pose:**

Sitting in the mountain pose, place your hands on your thighs and sit tall with your feet flat on the floor. As you ground yourself in the here and now, close your eyes and take a few deep breaths. Consider yourself to be a sturdy mountain. Feel your core's steadfastness and radiance of power. Hold this position for a little while while connecting to your inner source of life and energy.

- **Seated Cat-Cow Stretch:**

Sit at the edge of your chair with your feet hip-width apart to perform the seated cat-cow stretch. Take a big breath in, then, like a cat stretching, curve your spine as you exhale and tuck your chin into your chest. Repeatedly inhale, then, as you exhale, arch your back and raise your chest and chin to the sky like a cow stretching. Repetition of this fluid, smooth movement should be done while breathing normally. As you awaken, feel the energy moving through your spine.

- **Sun Salutation while seated:**

Sit tall with your feet flat on the floor. Take a deep breath in and raise your arms upward, reaching for the sky. Bring your hands to your heart's center as you exhale. As you exhale, fold forward and reach your hands toward the floor or your feet. Inhale, raising your arms back up. Take a deep breath in and raise your torso back up to your upright position. Repeat this flow of the sun salutations while seated several times, allowing your body and mind to be renewed by the movement and breath.

- **Twist and reach while seated:**

Sit up straight with your feet flat on the floor. Take a deep breath in and, as you let it out, twist your torso to the right, putting your right hand on the chair's backrest and your left hand on the outside of your right leg. Reaching as far as is comfortable, extend your left arm to the right side. For a few breaths, hold the twist while reaching, then come back to the center and repeat on the left side. This position boosts vigor and stimulates the flow of energy.

- **Breath of Fire when seated:**

Sit tall, with your feet flat on the floor, and place your hands on your thighs. Take a deep breath in, and start breathing quickly and rhythmically through your nose as you exhale. Keep the breaths constant in length, focusing on the sharp exhale. For 1-2 minutes, keep using the breath of fire technique while steadily increasing the intensity. The body and mind are energized by this breathing exercise, which enhances oxygen intake.

- **Standing Warrior Pose:**

Place your feet hip-width apart while sitting tall. Exhale while raising your right arm upward and moving it toward the left side. The right side of your body should feel longer. After a few breaths of holding, come back to your core. On the left, repeat. The body is given energy in this position, which heightens vitality.

- **Seated Lion's Breath:**

With your feet flat on the floor and your hands resting on your thighs, perform the seated lion's breath. Inhale deeply through your nose, then let out a lion's roar by opening your mouth wide and sticking out your tongue. Release any tension and boost your energy by performing the lion's breath practice three to five times.

You may increase your energy and revitalize your body and mind by incorporating these chair yoga poses and breathing exercises into your everyday routine. As you do things, be attentive to your requirements and those of your body. We shall discuss chair yoga for relaxation and stress reduction in the following chapter.

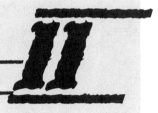

CHAPTER 11

CHAIR YOGA FOR STRESS REDUCTION

For seniors to enhance their general well-being and mental clarity, it is essential to find moments of relaxation and stress reduction. We'll look at a number of relaxing and stress-relieving chair yoga poses and practices in this chapter. You'll be able to relax, clear your mind, and find inner peace with the aid of these techniques.

- **Sitting Forward Fold:**

Keep your feet flat on the floor while sitting tall. Deeply inhale, then gently exhale while folding forward from the hips and reaching your hands toward the floor or your feet. Relax your neck and head by doing so. Hold this position for a few seconds while taking deep breaths and feeling your spine and back gently stretched. This position encourages relaxation and aids in the release of stress.

- **Seated Shoulder and Neck Release:**

Release your shoulders and neck while sitting upright with your feet flat on the floor. Take a deep breath in and, as you let it out, lower your right ear toward your right shoulder. You should feel a stretch along the left side of your neck. Hold for a few breaths, then come back to the middle and do it again, this time on the left side. Next, take a breath in and, as you exhale, lower your chin so that it stretches the back of your neck. After holding for a few breaths, slowly raise your head back up. This series facilitates relaxation by easing tension in the shoulders and neck.

- **Seated Heart Opener:**

Sit tall with your feet flat on the floor and clasp your hands behind your lower back for the seated heart opener. Deeply inhale, then softly elevate your chest and draw your shoulder blades together as you exhale. If it's comfortable, let your head slightly tilt back. Hold this position for a few seconds while taking deep breaths to open up the front of your body and encourage calm and openness.

- **Seated Side Stretch:**

Sit tall, your feet should be flat on the floor, and your arms should be raised aloft. Take a deep breath in and, as you exhale, slowly lean to the right until you feel your left side being stretched. Hold for a few breaths, then come back to the middle and do it again, this time on the left side. This position promotes relaxation and aids in the release of side-body tension.

- **Seated Butterfly Pose:**

Sit tall with your feet flat on the floor and bring the soles of your feet together while letting your knees fall out to the sides. This is the seated butterfly pose. For support, hold on to your shins or ankles. Deeply inhale, then, as you exhale, slowly lower your knees to the ground until you feel a stretch in your inner thighs and hips. Hold this position for a few moments while taking deep breaths, allowing yourself to unwind and let go of any tension.

- **Seated Meditation:**

Sit upright while meditating; your feet should be flat on the floor, and your hands should be relaxed against your thighs. Put your eyes closed and take a few slow, deep breaths. Pay close attention to your breathing and allow it to become even and relaxed. By letting go of your ideas and concerns, you can bring your focus to the present moment. Spend some time in this seated meditation, appreciating the calm and developing inner serenity.

- **Guided Relaxation Visualization:**

Close your eyes and take a comfortable seat. Put yourself in a serene setting, such as a lovely garden or a relaxing beach. Imagine the surroundings' sights, sounds, and sensations. Continue to inhale deeply, release any tension or stress, and allow yourself to completely lose yourself in this peaceful setting. Spend a few minutes in this guided visualization of relaxation and let yourself fall asleep.

To encourage relaxation, lower stress, and improve your general well-being, incorporate these chair yoga poses and relaxation practices into your everyday routine. Keep in mind to pay attention to your body, proceed at your own pace, and savor the peaceful moments. We shall discuss chair yoga for balance and coordination in the following chapter.

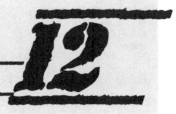

CHAIR YOGA FOR BALANCE AND COORDINATION

Seniors must maintain their balance and coordination to avoid falls and maintain their independence in daily activities. In this chapter, we'll look at several chair yoga poses and drills that are designed to increase balance and coordination. Your stability will rise, your proprioception will get better, and your core will get stronger with these exercises.

- **Sitting Tall with Flat Feet:**

Sit tall with flat feet. Lift your right leg off the ground while keeping it straight with your arms extended in front of you. Find your equilibrium by contracting your core and holding this position for a few breaths. Lower your right leg gradually, then do the same with your left. This pose develops the abdominal muscles and enhances stability and balance.

- **Seated Leg Cross:**

Sit tall, place your hands on your thighs, and keep your feet flat on the floor. Take a big breath in, and then, as you let it out, lift your right foot off the floor and cross it over your left leg, putting your right ankle on your left knee. In order to protect your knee, flex your right foot. Feel the stretch in your hips and thighs as you hold this position for a few breaths. On the opposite side, repeat. Balance and hip stability are enhanced in this stance.

- **Sitting Figure-Four Stretch:**

Keep your feet flat on the floor while sitting tall. Forming a figure-four, place your right ankle on top of your left leg. In order to protect your knee, flex your right foot. Deeply inhale, then, as you exhale, slowly lower your right knee to the ground until your hip and outer thigh are stretched. After a few breaths of holding this stretch, switch to the opposite side. Balance and hip stability are improved in this stance.

- **Seated Tree Pose:**

With your feet planted firmly on the ground, strike the "seated tree pose." Deeply inhale, and as you exhale, lift your right foot off the floor and, depending on your comfort level and balance, rest the right foot's sole against the inner of your left calf or thigh. Engage your core while pressing your foot into your leg. In order to maintain balance, find a focus point to look at. Repeat on the other side after holding the position for a few breaths. This position strengthens the leg muscles and enhances balance.

- **Seated Heel-to-Toe Stretch:**

Sit tall with your feet flat on the floor and your hands resting on your thighs while you perform a seated heel-to-toe stretch. Take a deep breath in, and then, as you exhale, lift your right foot off the floor and connect your right heel with your left toes. Hold your body in an upright stance for a few breaths. On the opposite side, repeat. This position enhances balance and coordination.

- **Eagle Arms when seated:**

Stand tall with your feet flat on the floor. Put your arms out in front at shoulder level. Bring your hands together or grasp onto the shoulders of the other person as you cross your right arm over your left arm. Your upper back and shoulders will stretch when you lift your elbows just a little. After a few breaths, hold this position and then alternate crossing your arms. This position strengthens the arms and shoulders while enhancing coordination.

- **Seated Swaying Palm Tree:**

With your feet flat on the ground and your hands resting on your thighs, assume the position of a standing, swaying palm tree. Deeply inhale, and as you exhale, gently rock your upper body side to side while letting your arms hang loose. Consider that you are a palm tree swinging in the wind. For a few breaths, continue this swaying motion, feeling the smooth flow and enhancing your sense of balance.

Improve your balance and coordination by including these chair yoga poses and exercises in your program.

Practice each position slowly and deliberately to establish stability. You will feel more assured in your movements and be able to maintain greater balance throughout your regular activities as you develop strength and coordination. We shall discuss chair yoga for flexibility and joint mobility in the following chapter.

CHAPTER 13

CHAIR YOGA FOR JOINT MOBILITY AND FLEXIBILITY

Seniors must maintain their flexibility and joint mobility in order to move freely and avoid stiffness. This chapter will go through several stretches and poses from chair yoga that are intended to increase flexibility and joint range of motion. These exercises can help you become more flexible overall, reduce tension in your muscles, and support joint health.

- **Seated Neck Stretch:**

Sit tall and stretch your neck while placing your hands on your thighs and your feet flat on the floor. Taking a deep breath in, slowly lower your right ear toward your right shoulder as you exhale. You should feel a stretch along the left side of your neck. Hold for a few breaths, then come back to the middle and do it again, this time on the left side. This stretch increases flexibility and relieves neck stress.

- **Seated Chest Opener:**

Sit tall, flat-footed, and interlace your hands behind your lower back. Deeply inhale, then softly elevate your chest and draw your shoulder blades together as you exhale. If it's comfortable, let your head slightly tilt back. Hold this position for a few moments while taking deep breaths and feeling the chest and shoulders stretch. This position encourages better posture and increases chest flexibility.

- **Sitting Forward Bend:**

Maintain a straight back and flat feet. Breathe deeply, then slowly tilt forward from your hips while reaching your hands toward the floor or your feet. Relax your neck and head by doing so. Hold this position for a few seconds while taking deep breaths and feeling your spine and back gently stretched. This stretch increases hamstring flexibility and eases lower back stress.

- **Seated Hip Opener:**

Sit tall and place your feet firmly on the ground for this seated hip opener. Allow your right knee to drift out to the side as you cross your right ankle across your left leg. To extend the stretch in your hip, softly press down on your right knee while maintaining a straight back. After holding for a few breaths, switch to the opposite side. This position eases stress on the hips and glutes and increases hip flexibility.

- **Sitting Spinal Twist:**

Ensure that your feet are planted firmly on the ground. Take a deep breath in and gradually twist your torso to the right as you exhale, placing your right hand on the chair's backrest and your left hand on the outside of your right leg. Take a few breaths while holding the twist while you look over your right shoulder. Repeat on the left side after exhaling to return to the center. This position stretches the back muscles and enhances spinal mobility.

- **Seated Ankle Circles:**

Sit tall and place your feet flat on the floor for the seated ankle circles. Lift your right foot off the ground and start rotating your ankle clockwise in a circle. Turn clockwise after 5–10 rounds, then counterclockwise. On the left, repeat. This exercise strengthens ankle and foot flexibility and enhances ankle mobility.

- **Seated Butterfly Stretch:**

Sit tall and place your feet flat on the floor for the seated butterfly stretch. Your knees should be free to sag out to the sides as you bring the soles of your feet together. For support, hold on to your shins or ankles. Deeply inhale, then, as you exhale, slowly lower your knees to the ground until you feel a stretch in your inner thighs and hips. Hold this stretch for a few breaths while taking deep breaths, allowing your hips and groin to loosen up and become more flexible.

To increase flexibility and joint mobility, incorporate these chair yoga poses and stretches into your everyday practice. Keep in mind to proceed slowly and in accordance with your current level of flexibility. You will experience more range of motion and ease in your motions as you keep practicing. We shall discuss chair yoga for energy and vigor in the following chapter.

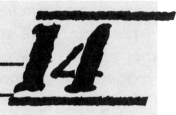

CHAIR YOGA FOR ENERGY AND VITALITY

For seniors to maintain an active lifestyle and take pleasure in their everyday activities, they must feel energized and alive. In this chapter, we'll look at a number of chair yoga poses and exercises with the goal of enhancing vitality and boosting energy. These exercises will assist in waking up your body, boosting circulation, and energizing your senses.

- **Seated Mountain Pose:**

Sitting in the mountain pose, place your hands on your thighs and sit tall with your feet flat on the floor. As you ground yourself in the here and now, close your eyes and take a few deep breaths. Think of yourself as a tall, stable mountain that is anchored and powerful. Imagine the life force reviving your entire body as it rises up from the earth via your spine. Spend a few seconds in this position while feeling stable and energized.

- **Seated Cat-Cow Stretch:**

Sit tall with your feet flat on the floor and your hands resting on your thighs for the seated cat-cow stretch. As you exhale, curve your spine and tuck your chin in toward your chest like a cat stretching. Take a big breath feet flat on the floor and your hands resting on your thighs for the seated cat-cow stretch. As you exhale, curve your spine and tuck your chin in toward your chest like a cat stretching. Take a big breath. Take a second breath in, and exhale while arching your back and lifting your chest forward like a cow. Replicate this fluid motion while synchronizing your breath. The spine is energized, and energy flow is increased by this stretch.

- **Sun Salutation while seated:**

Sit tall, place your feet flat on the floor, and place your hands on your thighs. Sweep your arms out to the sides and overhead, reaching up toward the sky, while you inhale. Bring your palms together in front of your heart as you inhale and feel the energy and warmth between them. Repeat this motion while breathing naturally. Imagine your entire existence being rejuvenated as you soak up the sun's vitality.

- **Seated Warrior Pose:**

With your feet flat on the floor and your hands resting on your thighs, strike the seated warrior pose. Exhale while raising your right arm aloft and leaning to the left. You should feel a stretch down the right side of your body. As you channel the strength and power within you, picture yourself as a brave and strong warrior. Repeat on the other side after inhaling to return to the center. Energy is increased, and a sense of assurance is fostered by this position.

- **Twist while seated:**

Sit tall, with your feet flat on the floor, and place your hands on your thighs. Take a deep breath in and, as you let it out, twist your torso to the right, putting your right hand on the chair's backrest and your left hand on the outside of your right leg. Then, hold the twist for a few breaths while taking a gentle look over your right shoulder. Repeat on the left side after inhaling to return to the center. This posture improves energy flow while stimulating the spine.

- **Breath of Fire when seated:**

Sit tall, with your feet flat on the floor, and place your hands on your thighs. Take a deep breath in and start rhythmically and firmly forcing air out of your nostrils. Allow your belly to softly contract with each exhalation, and allow your inhalations to happen naturally. Feel the burst of energy and vitality in your body as you hold this quick inhalation for 30 to 60 seconds. This breathing technique raises energy levels and oxygen intake.

- **Sitting Energizing Meditation:**

Take a comfortable seat and close your eyes. Breathe in vitality and exhale any exhaustion or tension as you take a few deep breaths. Imagine bright, vivacious energy flooding your body with vigor with each inhalation.

Visualize any stuck or stagnant energy leaving your body with each breath to make room for new energy to flow. Spend a few minutes in this energizing meditation, feeling refreshed and renewed.

To increase your energy levels and encourage a sense of vigor, incorporate these chair yoga positions and practices into your daily schedule. Keep in mind that you should respect the limitations and needs of your body. You'll have more energy, a sharper focus, and a greater enthusiasm for life if you develop a regular practice. We'll give you a 10-week training schedule with detailed illustrations in the last chapter to make it easier for you to successfully incorporate these chair yoga techniques into your daily life.

CHAPTER 15

CHAIR YOGA TRAINING PROGRAM FOR TEN WEEKS

A 10-week chair yoga training schedule for seniors over 60 is provided below, along with detailed illustrations of how to perform each exercise:

WEEK ONE: WELCOME AND FOUNDATIONAL MOVEMENTS

DAY — 1:

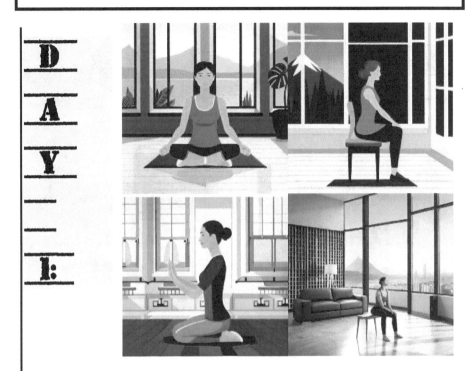

1. Sit tall on a chair in the mountain pose with your feet flat on the floor and your hands resting on your thighs. Take a few deep breaths, relax, and close your eyes.

2. Fold forward when seated by hinging from the hips and extending your arms down to your feet. Pause between breaths.

3. Seated rotation: Sit tall and gradually rotate your upper body to the right while placing your left palm on the outside of your right leg. Hold for a few breaths, then switch to the opposite side.

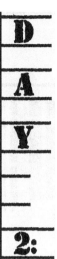

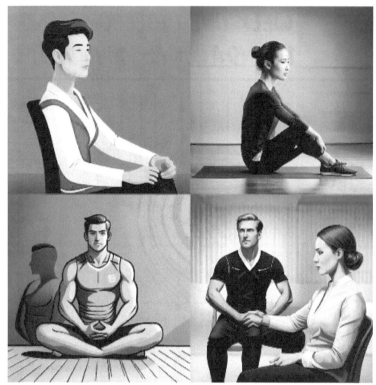

1. Seated Shoulder Rolls: Roll your shoulders in a circular motion while sitting tall. Repeat 5 to 8 times.

2. Stretching the neck while seated involves lowering the right ear toward the right shoulder, holding the position for a few breaths, then switching to the opposite side. Next, hold as you droop your chin toward your chest. Lastly, raise your head and look up at the ceiling.

3. Interlace your fingers behind your back, push your shoulder blades together, and elevate your chest while seated to open your chest. Pause between breaths.

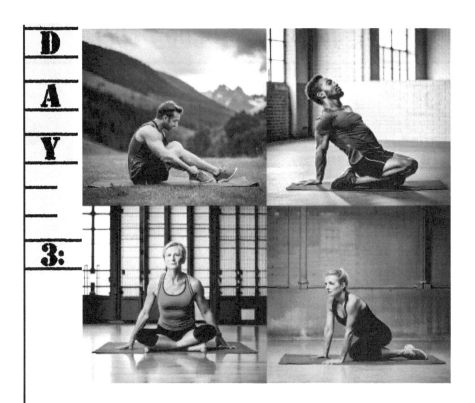

1. Position your hands on your knees, curve your back like a cat while breathing, and then arch it upward while inhaling in the seated cat-cow position. For a few rounds, keep doing this motion while synchronizing it with your breathing.

2. Sit up straight, lift one leg toward your chest, hold it for a second, and then lower it. For a few repetitions, alternate between the legs.

3. Sitting Ankle Rolls: Extend one leg, roll your ankle in a circle, and then change the angle of the rotation. Continue with the opposite leg.

WEEK TWO: UPPER BODY FOCUS

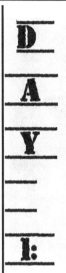

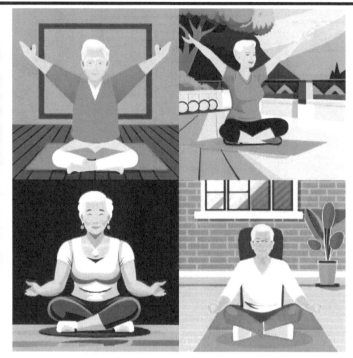

1. Circles made with the arms while seated: Extend your arms out to the sides. Increase the size of the circles gradually before turning around.

2. Stretch your chest while seated by clapping your hands behind your back, keeping your arms straight. Pause between breaths.

3. Stretching the triceps while seated involves raising one arm overhead, bending the elbow, and reaching the other shoulder blade with the hand. With your other hand, gently press the elbow. After a few breaths of holding, switch sides.

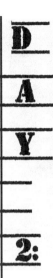

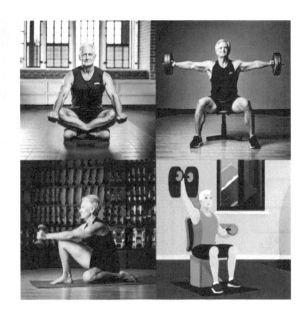

1. Hold a small dumbbell or water bottle in each hand while performing seated bicep curls. Bring the weights nearer to your shoulders while maintaining a tall posture and bent elbows. Reducing them once more. Repeat a couple of times more.

2. Hold a weight in each hand, starting at shoulder height, for the seated shoulder press. Lift your arms up, then bring them back down. Repeat a couple of times more.

3. Hold a weight in each hand while doing side raises while seated. Bring your arms parallel to the floor by raising them out to the sides. Reducing them once more. Repeat a couple of times more.

4. Stretch your wrists while seated by extending your arms in front of you with your palms down. Feel the stretch in your forearms as you gently bend your wrists upward and downward. Repeat several times.

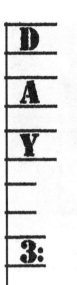

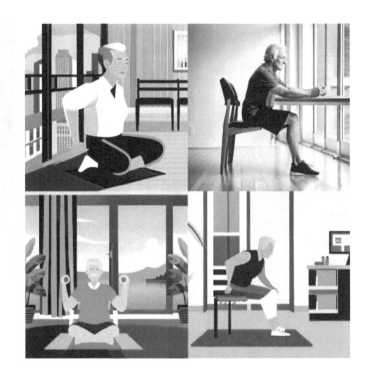

1. Put your hands shoulder-width apart on the edge of the chair and perform push-ups while seated. By bending your elbows, bring your chest close to the chair before pushing yourself back up. Repeat a couple times more.

2. Holding a weight in one hand, raising your arm overhead, and bending your elbow such that the weight is behind your head are all seated overhead tricep extensions. Straighten your elbow as you raise your arm. Reducing it once again. Repeat a few times, then swap sides.

3. Rows while seated: Sit up straight, grasp a towel or resistance band in front of you, and draw your hands in close to your body while pressing your shoulder blades together. After a few repetitions, release and repeat.

DAY 1:

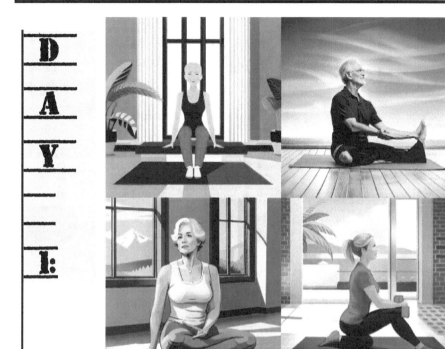

1. Sit tall, extend one leg forward, and hold the position for a few breaths. Repeat with the second leg after lowering it once more. Add ankle weights for an additional challenge.

2. Sit down and perform sitting calf raises by lifting your heels off the floor and rising to your toes. Reducing them once more. Repeat a couple of times more.

3. Sitting Heel Lifts: Sitting, lift your toes off the floor while maintaining your heels on the floor. Reducing them once more. Repeat a couple of times more.

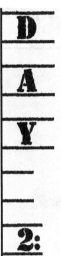

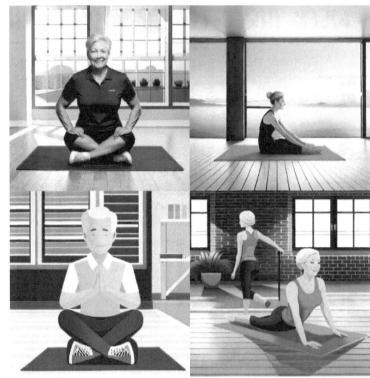

1. Knee-to-Chest Stretch While Seated: Sit up straight, bring one knee up to your chest, and hold for a few breaths. Repeat with the other leg after releasing.

2. Stretch your hamstrings while seated by leaning forward from your hips while sitting on the edge of the chair and extending one leg. Feel the stretch in your leg's back. After a few breaths of holding, switch sides.

3. Stretching your quads while sitting up straight, bending one leg, and bringing your foot toward your glutes gently press your foot into your hand while holding it in place. After a few breaths, hold and switch to the other leg.

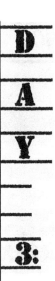

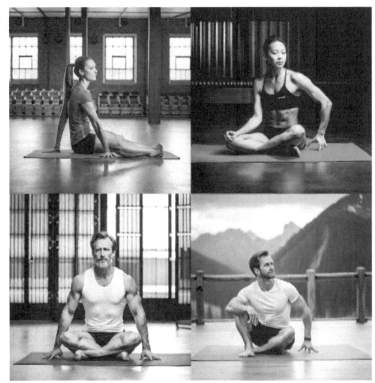

1. Sit tall, cross one ankle over the other knee, and gently press down on the raised knee to perform the seated Figure Four Stretch. Feel the hip being stretched. After a few breaths of holding, switch sides.

2. Butterfly stretch while seated: Sit tall, bring your feet close together, and slowly lower your knees to the floor. Pause between breaths.

3. Sun Salutations while seated: Begin in Mountain Pose while seated, lift your arms aloft, and then bring them down to your heart. Repeat many times while synchronizing your breath.

WEEK FOUR: STABILITY AND BALANCE

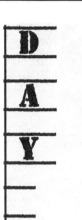

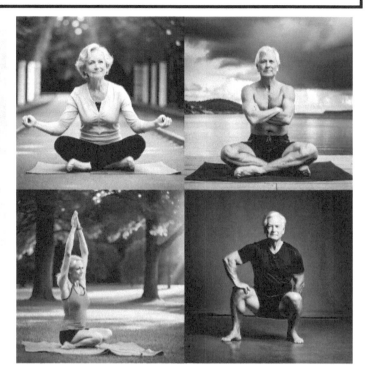

1. In the seated Eagle Pose, bring your palms together, cross one leg over the other, and wrap the other arm across the other. After a few breaths of holding, switch sides.

2. Find your balance in the tree pose while seated by placing one foot on the inner thigh of the other leg. Put your hands in front of your heart in a prayer possessing one foot on the inner thigh of the other leg. Put your hands in front of your heart in a prayer pose. After a few breaths of holding, switch sides.

3. Chair Pose while seated: Sit tall, tense your abdomen, and raise your arms in the air. Pause between breaths.

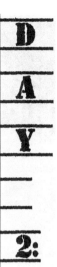

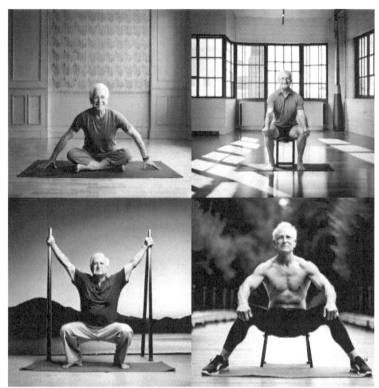

1. Put your hands on the chair's arms while standing in the seated bridge position with your feet flat on the floor and hip distance apart. Create a bridge-like form with your body by pressing through your feet and lifting your hips off the chair. Release after a brief period of holding.

2. Sitting Happy Baby Pose: Place your knees close to your chest and place your hands on the soles of your feet. Rock slowly from side to side.

3. Cross one ankle over the other knee while seated in pigeon pose. Flex the foot and softly press the knee down. After a few breaths of holding, switch sides.

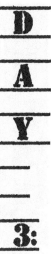

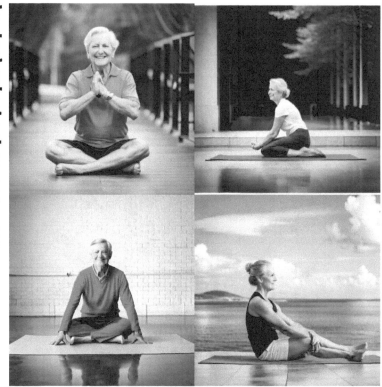

1. Child's Pose, while seated, involves bringing your knees wide, folding forward with your body resting between your thighs, and sitting closer to the front edge of the chair. Put your arms out in front of you or place them on the seat of the chair.

2. Seated Boat Pose: Elevate your legs off the floor while keeping your knees bent. Sit close to the front edge of the chair, lean back slightly, engage your core, and elevate your legs. Pause between breaths.

3. Sit tall, put your hands on the chair's arms, slowly arch your spine, and lift your chest in the seated sphinx position. Pause between breaths.

WEEK FIVE: MOBILITY AND FLEXIBILITY

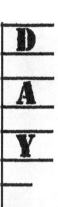

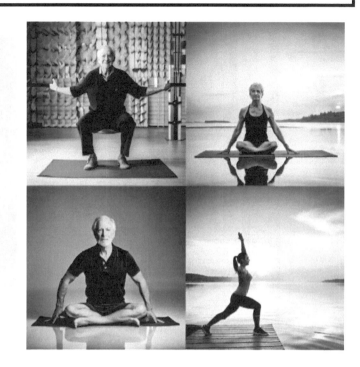

1. Stack one knee on top of the other while sitting tall in the cow-face position. Slide your feet out to the sides. Lifting your chest while tying your fingers together behind your back. After a few breaths of holding, switch sides.

2. Open your legs wide in the extended triangle pose while seated. Turn your right foot out, reach your right arm toward it, and raise your left arm toward the ceiling. After a few breaths of holding, switch sides.

3. Half Moon Pose when seated: Sit close to the front of the chair, slant your head to one side, and raise your arm overhead. Keep your core active for stability. After a few breaths of holding, switch sides.

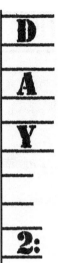

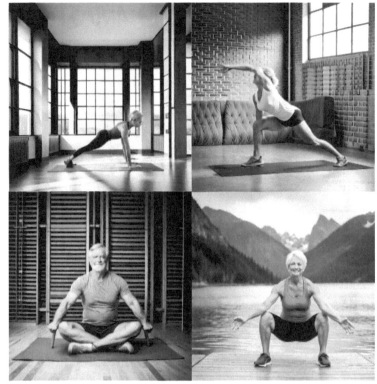

1. Side planking when seated is achieved by placing one hand on the chair's armrest, extending your legs out to the sides, and lifting your hips off the seat. After a few breaths of holding, switch sides.

2. Modified Camel Pose when seated: Sit close to the front edge of the chair, support your lower back with your hands, gently arch your spine, and lift your chest. Pause between breaths.

3. Seated Reclining Bound Angle Pose: Sit with your feet together, facing the front of the chair, and lean back, utilizing the chair's backrest as support. Pause between breaths.

DAY 3:

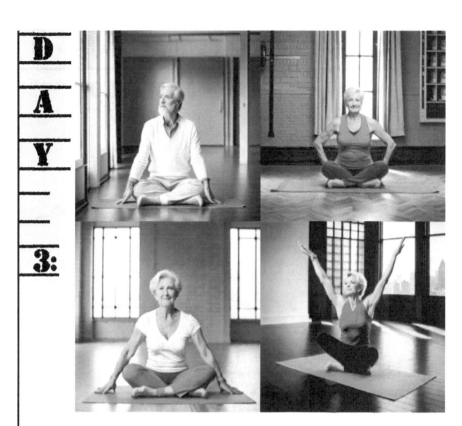

1. Twist your upper body gently to the opposite side while seated supine. Sit close to the front edge of the chair, cross one leg over the other, and do this position. After a few breaths of holding, switch sides.

2. Legs Up the Wall Pose: Place your legs up the wall while seated, resting them against the wall. Sit toward the front edge of the chair. Breathe deeply and let your body relax.

3. Butterfly Pose while seated: Sit close to the front edge of the chair, put your feet together, and lean back, utilizing the chair's backrest as support. Your knees should be free to fall open to the sides. Pause between breaths.

WEEK SIX: ENDURANCE AND STRENGTH

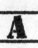

DAY 1:

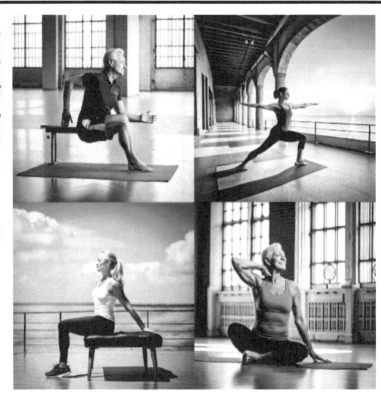

1. Sit tall, lay your hands on your lower back, slowly arch your spine, and lift your chest in the camel pose while seated. Pause between breaths.

2. Seated Locust Pose: Sit tall, reach your arms out in front of you, and lift both of your legs off the floor while maintaining them straight. Pause between breaths.

3. Bow Pose while seated: Sit tall, grip the chair's sides, lift your chest, and draw your shoulder blades together. Lift your feet off the ground if it's comfortable. Pause between breaths.

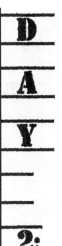

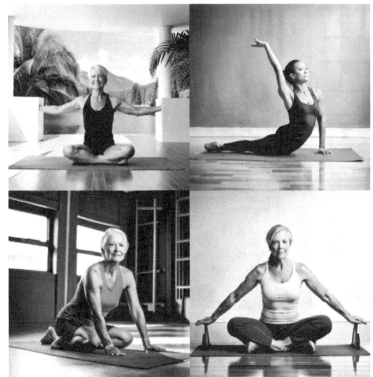

1. Seated Bridge Pose with Leg Lifts: Start in Seated Bridge Pose (Day 2 of Week 4), then lift one leg straight up to the ceiling. After a few breaths of holding, switch legs.

2. Seated Warrior III Pose: Sit tall, elevate your back leg, lean forward, stretch one leg, and reach your hands toward the floor. Find your equilibrium. After a few breaths of holding, switch legs.

3. Head-to-knee forward bends while seated: Sit tall, stretch one leg forward, and bend the other knee so that the sole of your foot touches the inner thigh of the forward-extending leg. Reaching toward your extended leg, bend forward. After a few breaths of holding, switch legs.

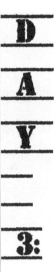

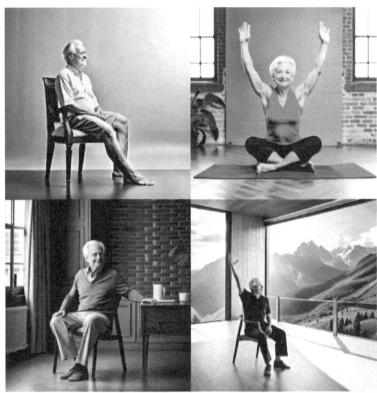

1. Hand-to-Big Toe Pose when Seated Reclining: Sit at the front edge of the chair, extend one leg forward, and place your hand on the big toe of that foot. Keep the leg straight as you raise it toward the ceiling. After a few breaths of holding, switch legs.

2. Seated Supported Shoulder Stand: Place your hands behind your lower back to support it while you sit near the front edge of the chair, lean back, and lift your legs overhead. Pause between breaths.

3. From the seated supported shoulder stand, take the seated plow pose by lowering your legs behind your head and pointing your toes downward. With your hands, support your back. Pause between breaths.

DAY 1:

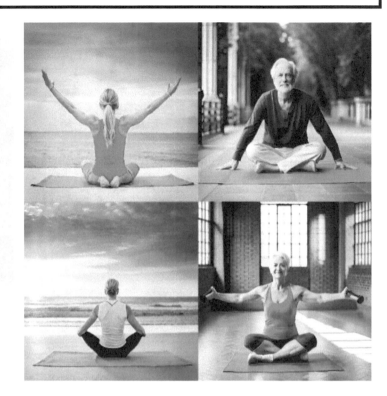

1. Relaxed Seated Forward Fold: Sit tall, hinge forward from the hips, and let your upper body dangle. Allow your arms to dangle while inhaling slowly and deeply. Pause between breaths.

2. In a seated position, roll your neck in a circular motion while maintaining a tall posture. After a few cycles, repeat in the other direction.

3. Seated Shoulder Release: Sit tall, cross one arm across your chest, and gently bring the arm in toward your body with the other hand. After a few breaths of holding, switch sides.

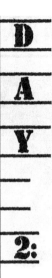

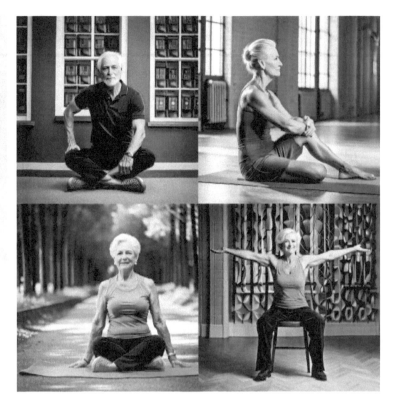

1. Variation of the seated twist with arms: Sit tall, place one hand on the chair's backrest, and gradually twist your upper body to the opposite side. The twist will be enhanced if you extend your other arm. After a few breaths of holding, switch sides.

2. Seated Side Bend: In order to create a stretch throughout your torso, sit tall, raise one arm above, and gently lean to the side. After a few breaths of holding, switch sides.

3. Sit tall, cross one ankle over the other knee, and gently press down on the lifted knee until you feel a stretch in your hip. This is a seated ankle-to-knee stretch. After a few breaths of holding, switch sides.

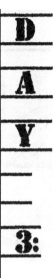

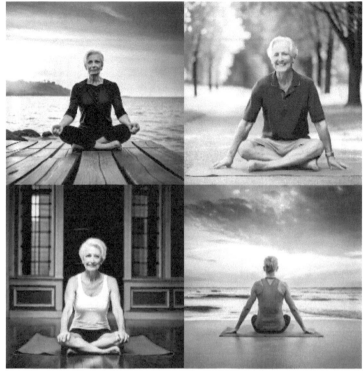

1. Sit tall, entwine your fingers behind your back, and elevate your chest to open your heart while you are seated. Pause between breaths.

2. Exercises for Seated Eyes: Sit up straight, relax your shoulders, and fix your sight on various areas of the room while gliding your eyes up, down, and side to side. Repeat several times.

3. Sit tall, close your eyes, and take a few slow, deep breaths while concentrating on how your breath feels entering and leaving your body. Spend a few minutes exercising.

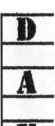

DAY 1:

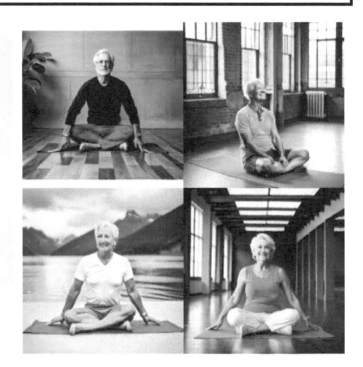

1. Seated Spinal Rotation: Sit tall, put your left hand on your right thigh outside, and slowly rotate your upper body to the right. Hold for a few breaths, then switch to the opposite side.

2. Knee-to-Elbow Crunches While Seated: Sit tall, raise one arm overhead, and crunch your body while bringing the opposing knee to your elbow. After a few repetitions, switch sides.

3. Sit tall, lean back slightly, elevate your feet off the floor, and perform seated Russian twists by swiveling your torso from side to side while touching the chair on each side. Repeat several times.

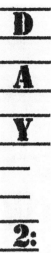

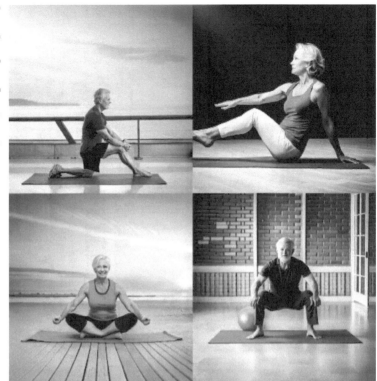

1. Plank posture while seated is achieved by sitting close to the front edge of the chair, resting your hands on the armrests, and stepping your feet back. Hold while contracting your core for a few breaths.

2. Leg Raises While Seated: Sit tall, extend one leg in front of you, and lift it off the floor while maintaining a straight leg. After a few breaths of holding, bring it back down. the other leg, and repeat.

3. Sit upright, put your hands behind your head, and perform seated bicycle crunches by bringing one knee up to your chest and rotating your body such that the opposite elbow touches the knee. After a few repetitions, switch sides.

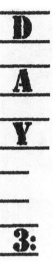

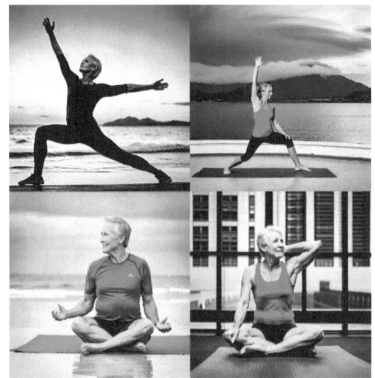

1. Sit tall, extend your legs forward, lift them off the floor, and balance on your sit bones in the seated boat pose with a twist. Turn your upper body to one side while bringing the opposing elbow up to the outside of your knee. After a few breaths of holding, switch sides.

2. Variation of the side plank while seated: Sit close to the front edge of the chair, lay one hand on the armrest, spread your legs out to the sides, and lift your hips off the seat to assume the position of the side plank. After a few breaths of holding, switch sides.

3. Sit tall, put your hands on the chair's seat, and alternately pull your knees to your chest as if you were sprinting in place for the exercise known as "seated mountain climbing." Keep going for several rounds.

WEEK NINE: MEDITATION AND MINDFULNESS

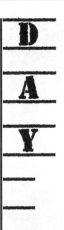

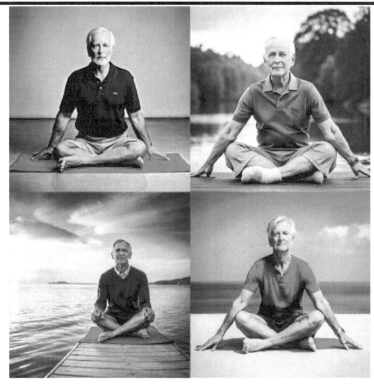

1. Sit upright, close your eyes, and concentrate on your breath when doing seated mindful breathing. Watch each breath in and out without attempting to alter it. Spend a few minutes exercising.

2. Specialize your eyes and perform a seated body scan by paying special attention to various body parts, beginning at your toes and working your way up to your head.

3. Consciously relax any tense or uncomfortable regions that you may have noticed.

DAY 2:

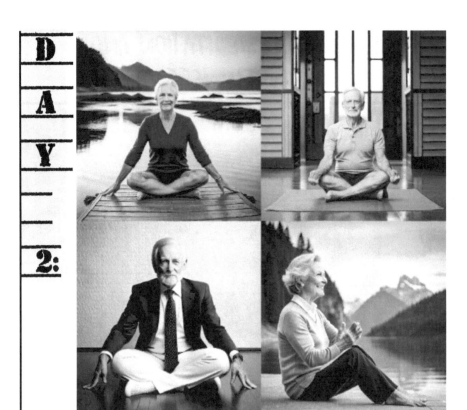

1. Guided meditation while seated: Select a guided meditation app or recording that meets your interests and follow along while relaxing in your chair. Any desired objective, such as relaxation or mindfulness, should be your main focus.

2. Choose a calming word or phrase that speaks to you, such as "peace" or "calm," then practice seated mantra meditation by sitting tall, closing your eyes, and silently repeating the mantra in your mind, allowing it to fill your awareness.

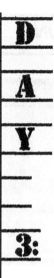

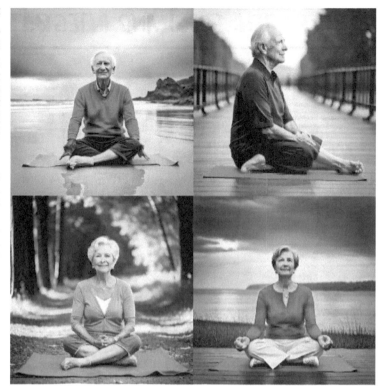

1. Sit tall, close your eyes, and think of a loved one during this seated loving-kindness meditation. Extend loving-kindness to yourself, a neutral person, and ultimately to all beings by repeating statements like "May you be happy. May you be healthy. May you live with ease."

2. Seated Gratitude Exercise: Close your eyes, sit up straight, and list three things for which you are thankful.

3. Develop an attitude of appreciation and let thankfulness overflow from your heart.

WEEK TEN: FLOW AND INTEGRATION

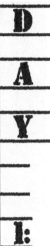

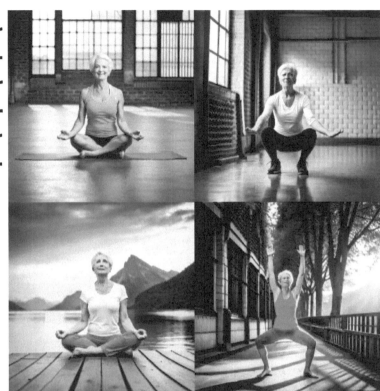

1. Sun Salutations while seated: Begin in Mountain Pose while seated, lift your arms aloft, and then bring them down to your heart. Repeat many times while synchronizing your breath.

2. Seated Flowing Cat-Cow: Sit tall, put your hands on your thighs, and round and arch your spine alternately like a cat and a cow.

3. Synchronize your breath with the two movements as you travel between them.

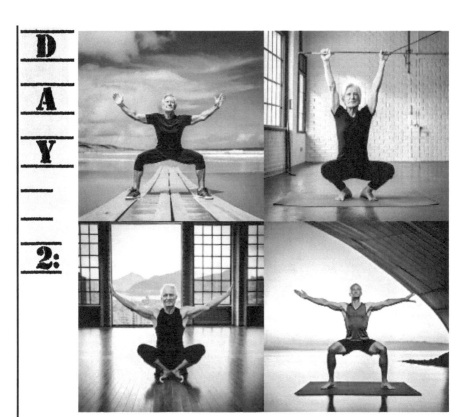

1. Sequence of the Seated Warrior: Sit tall, elevate your rear leg, extend one leg forward, lean forward, and reach your hands to the floor.

2. Straighten your back leg and extend your arms forward to move into Seated Warrior III.

3. Bend your back leg and lift your arms overhead to return to Seated Warrior I. On the opposite side, repeat.

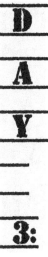

DAY 3:

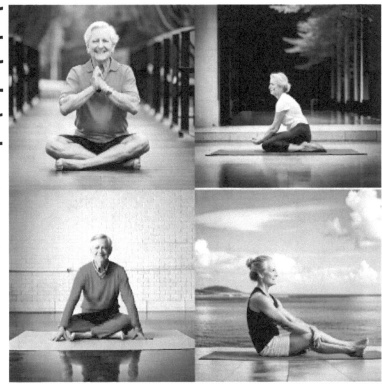

1. Sit tall, extend one leg to the side, reach your arm aloft, and bend to the opposite side to perform the seated Flowing Half Moon.

2. Move between the two sides while breathing deeply and letting your body settle into a soothing rhythm.

Congratulations on finishing the chair yoga training program after 10 weeks! Always pay attention to your body, adjust any positions as necessary, and reap the rewards of your yoga practice.

CONCLUSION

For seniors over 60, chair yoga is an excellent and convenient type of exercise that has many psychological, emotional, and physical advantages. We have examined the tenets, methods, and postures of chair yoga throughout this manual to give seniors a thorough starting point for their yoga journey.

Seniors can achieve increases in flexibility, strength, balance, and general well-being by practicing chair yoga on a daily basis. For people with physical limitations or restricted mobility, chair yoga is the perfect option due to its gentle nature, which enables them to experience the health benefits of yoga while still feeling at ease in their seats.

The versatility of chair yoga is one of its main benefits. A safe and pleasurable practice is guaranteed by the ability to modify each position to meet unique requirements and skills. Seniors can customize their practice to their own needs by altering the range of motion, utilizing props for support, or taking breaks as necessary, making it accessible and appropriate for all fitness levels.

In addition to its physical advantages, chair yoga promotes mental and emotional health. Stress reduction, mental clarity, and an inner sense of peace are encouraged through an emphasis on mindful breathing, meditation, and relaxation exercises. Seniors who practice chair yoga can find comfort in it, which enables them to relax, develop self-awareness, and improve their general quality of life.

Chair yoga also promotes interpersonal interaction and civic participation. Seniors who practice chair yoga or take sessions with others might develop a sense of community and support. It gives people a chance to talk, exchange stories, and form connections, preventing social isolation and fostering a sense of community.

As with any workout regimen, seniors should speak with their doctors before beginning chair yoga, especially if they have any underlying medical issues. Seniors should also pace themselves and make adjustments as needed, paying attention to their bodies. Since every person's path will be different, it is essential to put safety and self-care first throughout the practice.

In conclusion, chair yoga is an excellent way for seniors over 60 to practice a comprehensive and enriching workout regimen. Seniors can improve their well-being, keep their independence, and age gracefully thanks to the wealth of physical, mental, and emotional advantages it offers. Seniors who practice chair yoga can benefit from its transforming abilities and cultivate a balance between their minds, body, and soul.

Made in United States
Troutdale, OR
09/29/2023

13278846R00056